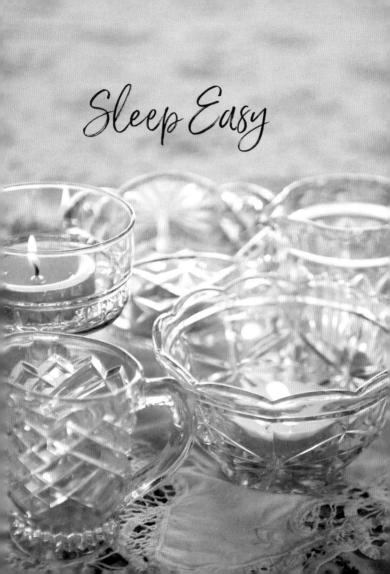

Sleep Easy

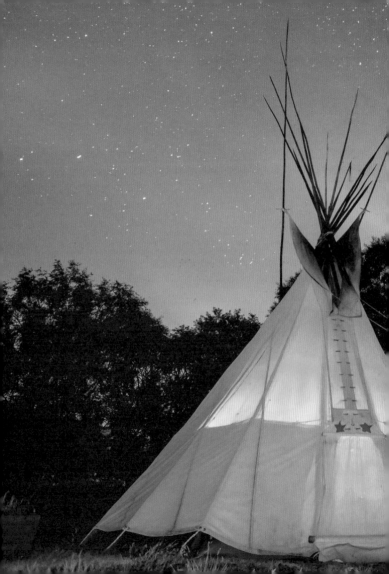

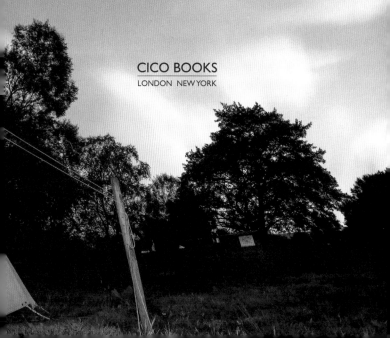

Sleep Easy

Soothing mantras and inspiration for
peace, calm, and a good night's rest

CICO BOOKS
LONDON NEW YORK

This edition published in 2025 by CICO Books
An imprint of Ryland Peters & Small Ltd
20–21 Jockey's Fields   1452 Davis Bugg Road
London WC1R 4BW   Warrenton, NC 27589

www.rylandpeters.com

10 9 8 7 6 5 4 3 2 1

First published in 2017 as *Evening Mantras*

Design © CICO Books 2017, 2025

For photography credits, see pages 143–144.

A CIP catalog record for this book is available from
the Library of Congress and the British Library.

ISBN: 978-1-80065-413-6

Printed in China

Commissioning editor: Kristine Pidkameny
Senior editor: Carmel Edmonds
Design concept: Paul Tilby
Designer: Geoff Borin
Art director: Sally Powell
Creative director: Leslie Harrington
Head of production: Patricia Harrington
Publishing manager: Penny Craig
Publisher: Cindy Richards

INTRODUCTION

Ending your day well is key to a better night's sleep. Within this book you will find a collection of carefully selected and beautifully presented words, mantras, and quotations. Each one will enable you to set your mind at ease, leaving you ready for rest and peaceful dreams.

Some mantras are helpful reminders to take the time to relax so you feel restored from the day's activities. Others encourage you to wonder more and worry less. The words of wisdom here guide you to nurture and find balance in your relationships, not only with family and friends, but also with yourself.

You can use these mantras in a number of ways. You may wish to read one every night, perhaps at the start of the evening when you need a new perspective, or right before going to bed so the thought stays with you while you sleep. Try writing down your favorites in a journal, or on cards to keep on a nightstand or maybe to put under your pillow. You could even send them to friends or family for inspiration.

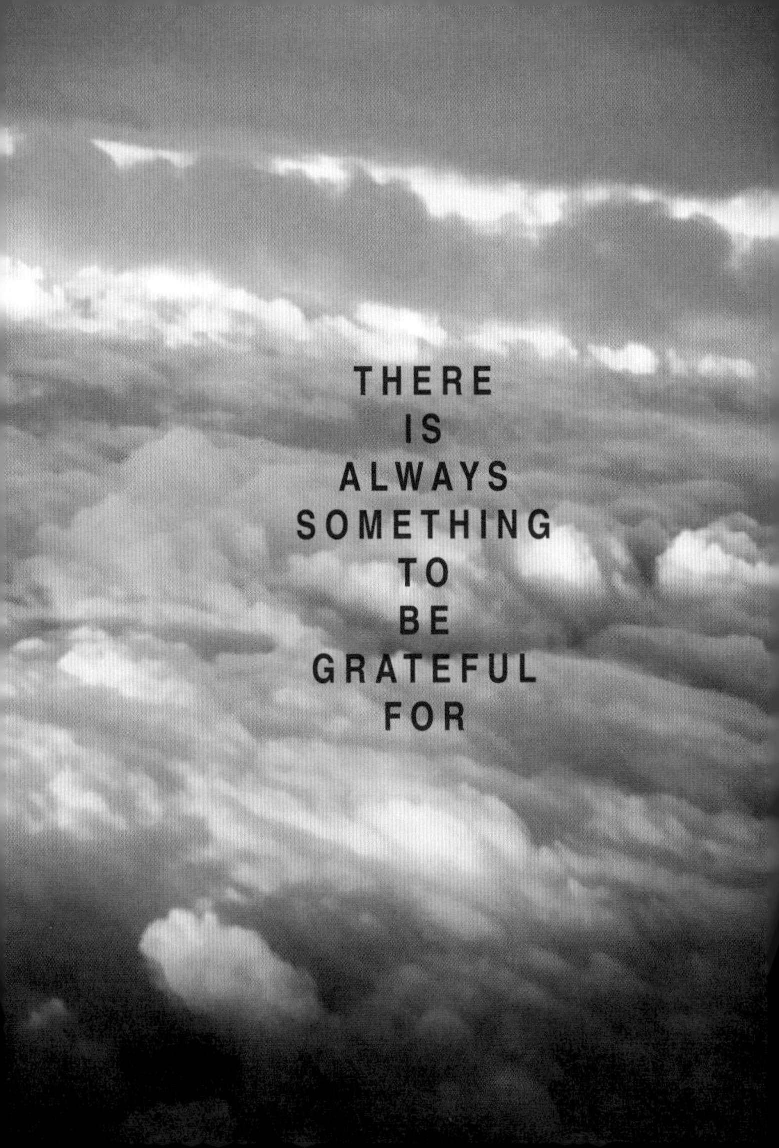

THERE
IS
ALWAYS
SOMETHING
TO
BE
GRATEFUL
FOR

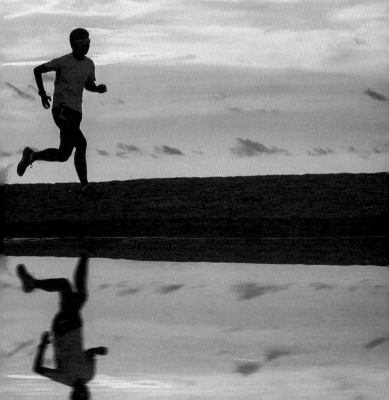

BE TRUTHFUL, GENTLE,
AND FEARLESS

ALL SHALL BE WELL, AND ALL SHALL BE WELL, AND ALL MANNER OF THINGS SHALL BE WELL

Julian of Norwich

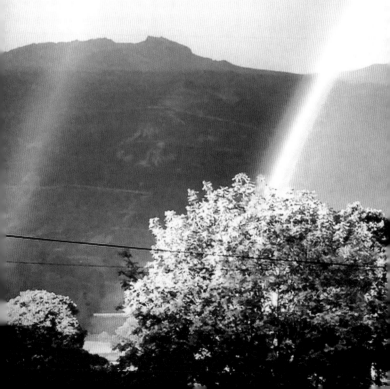

WHAT WE THINK, WE BECOME

Buddha

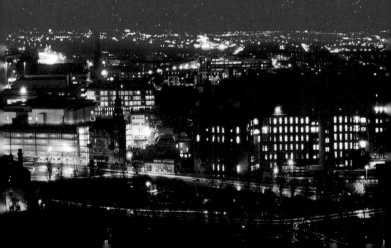

I KNOW NOTHING
WITH ANY CERTAINTY,
BUT THE SIGHT OF STARS
MAKES ME DREAM

Vincent van Gogh

BE THE SPARK, ESPECIALLY
WHEN IT'S DARK

IF THE ONLY PRAYER YOU
EVER SAY IN YOUR ENTIRE
LIFE IS THANK YOU,
IT WILL BE ENOUGH

Meister Eckhart

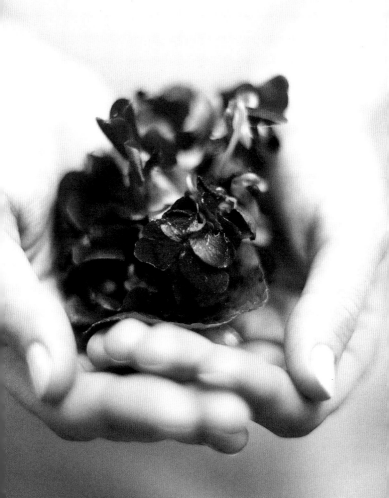

TAKE REST:

A FIELD THAT HAS
RESTED GIVES A
BEAUTIFUL CROP

Ovid

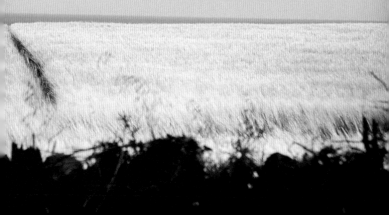

PUT YOUR THOUGHTS TO SLEEP,
DO NOT LET THEM CAST A SHADOW
OVER THE MOON OF YOUR HEART.
LET GO OF THINKING

Rumi

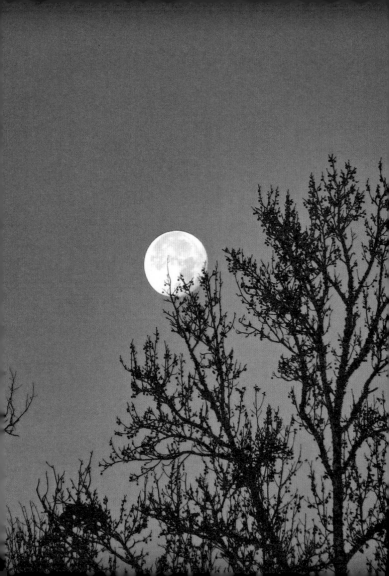

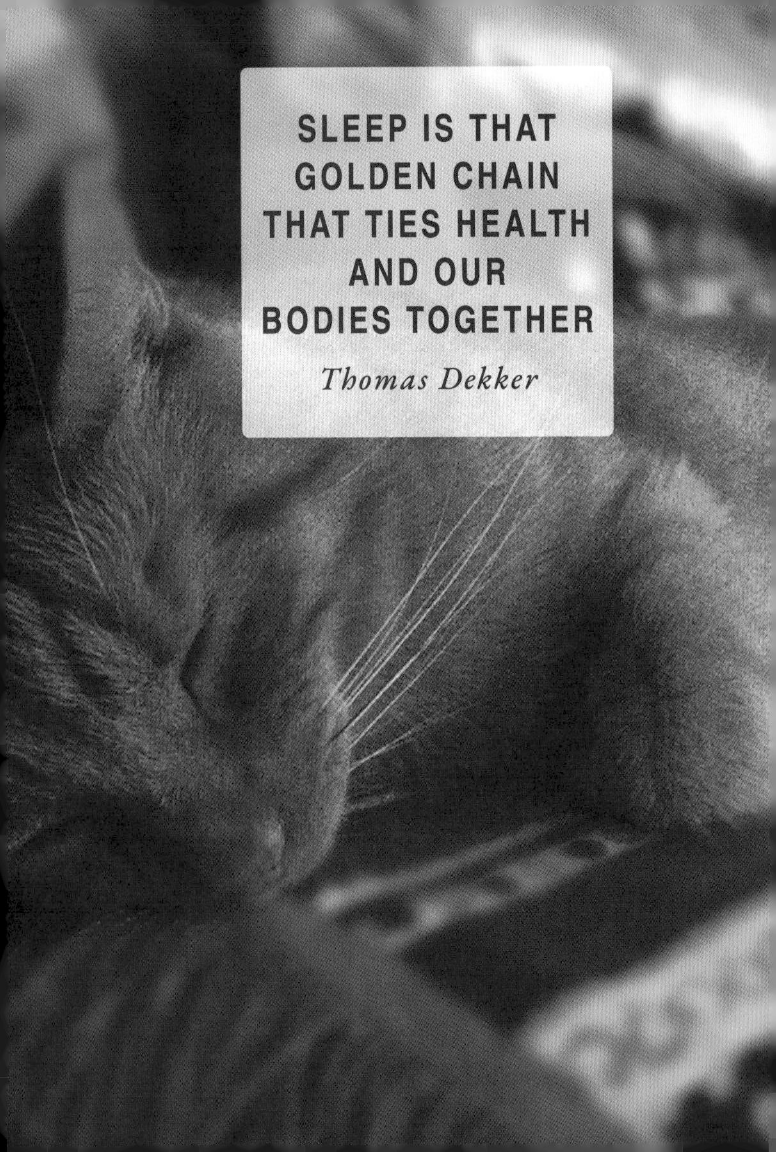

SLEEP IS THAT
GOLDEN CHAIN
THAT TIES HEALTH
AND OUR
BODIES TOGETHER

Thomas Dekker

CONNECT WITH YOUR DIVINE SOURCE

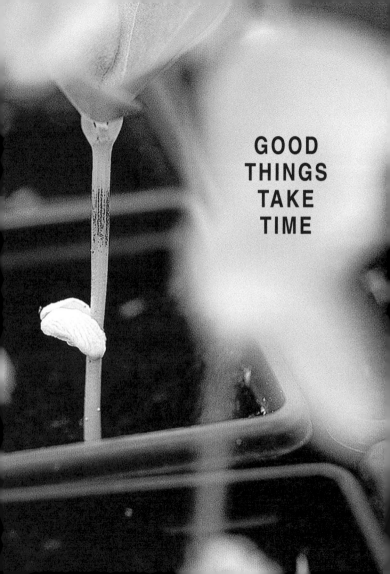

GOOD
THINGS
TAKE
TIME

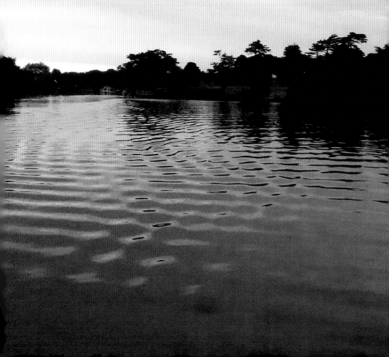

WE DO NOT LEARN
FROM EXPERIENCE ... WE
LEARN FROM REFLECTING
ON EXPERIENCE

UNPLUG

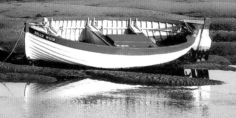

WORRYING WILL NEVER CHANGE THE OUTCOME

LET IT GO

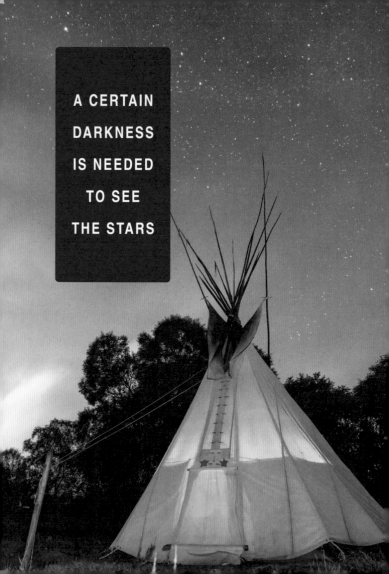

A CERTAIN DARKNESS IS NEEDED TO SEE THE STARS

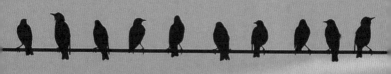

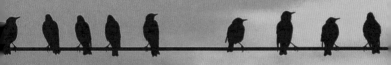

ONCE YOU MAKE A DECISION, THE UNIVERSE CONSPIRES TO MAKE IT HAPPEN

Ralph Waldo Emerson

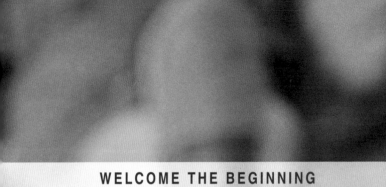

**WELCOME THE BEGINNING
OF A NEW EVENING**

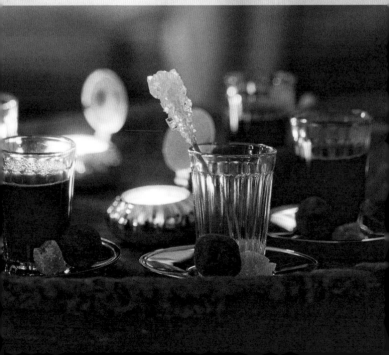

DELIGHT AT THE PROMISE
OF A NEW TOMORROW

VERY LITTLE IS NEEDED TO MAKE A HAPPY LIFE; IT IS ALL WITHIN YOURSELF, IN YOUR WAY OF THINKING

Marcus Aurelius

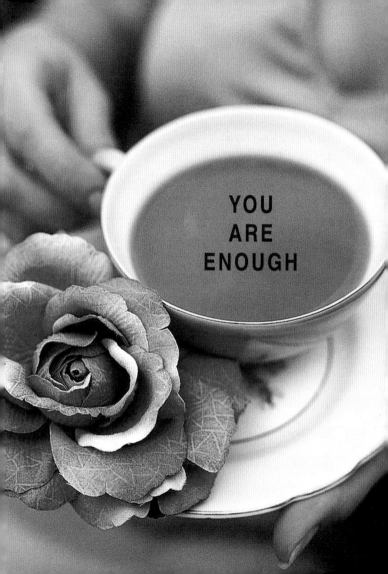

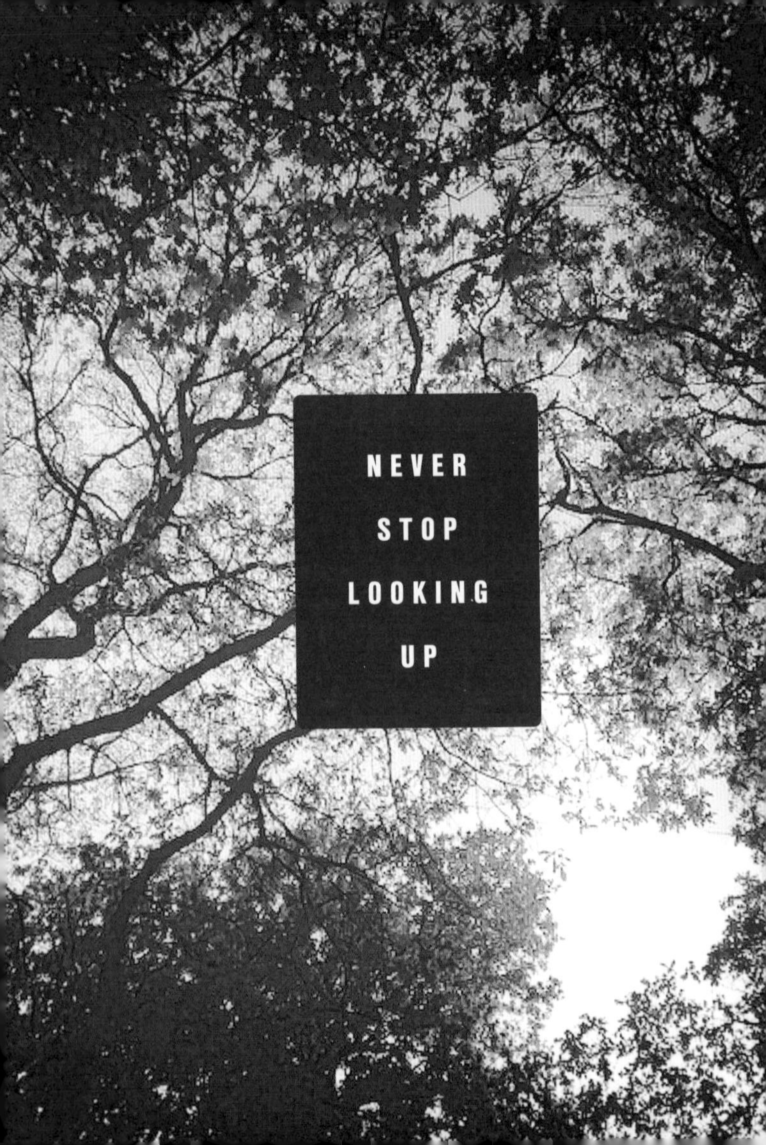

NEVER

STOP

LOOKING

UP

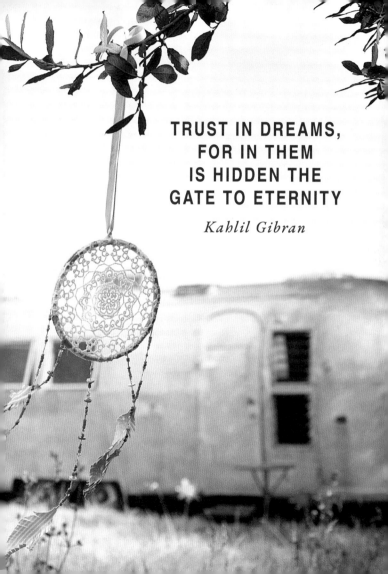

**TRUST IN DREAMS,
FOR IN THEM
IS HIDDEN THE
GATE TO ETERNITY**

Kahlil Gibran

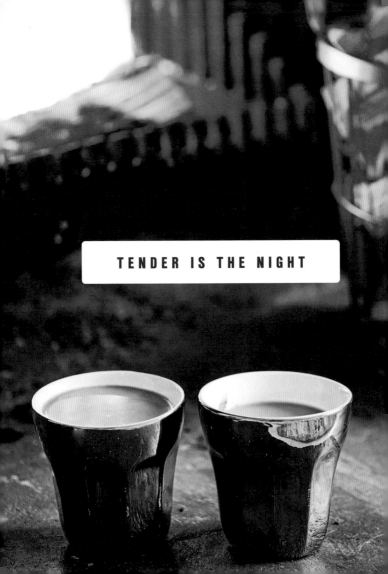

TENDER IS THE NIGHT

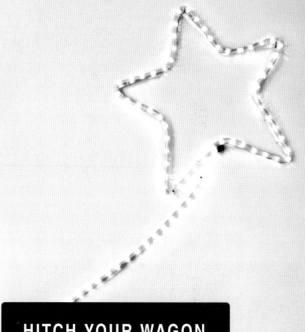

HITCH YOUR WAGON
TO A STAR

Ralph Waldo Emerson

If a little dreaming

is dangerous, the cure for

it is not to dream less but

to dream more, to dream

all the time

Marcel Proust

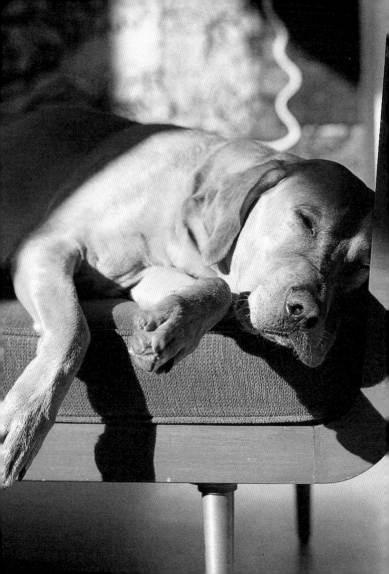

WHAT YOU SEEK
IS SEEKING YOU

Rumi

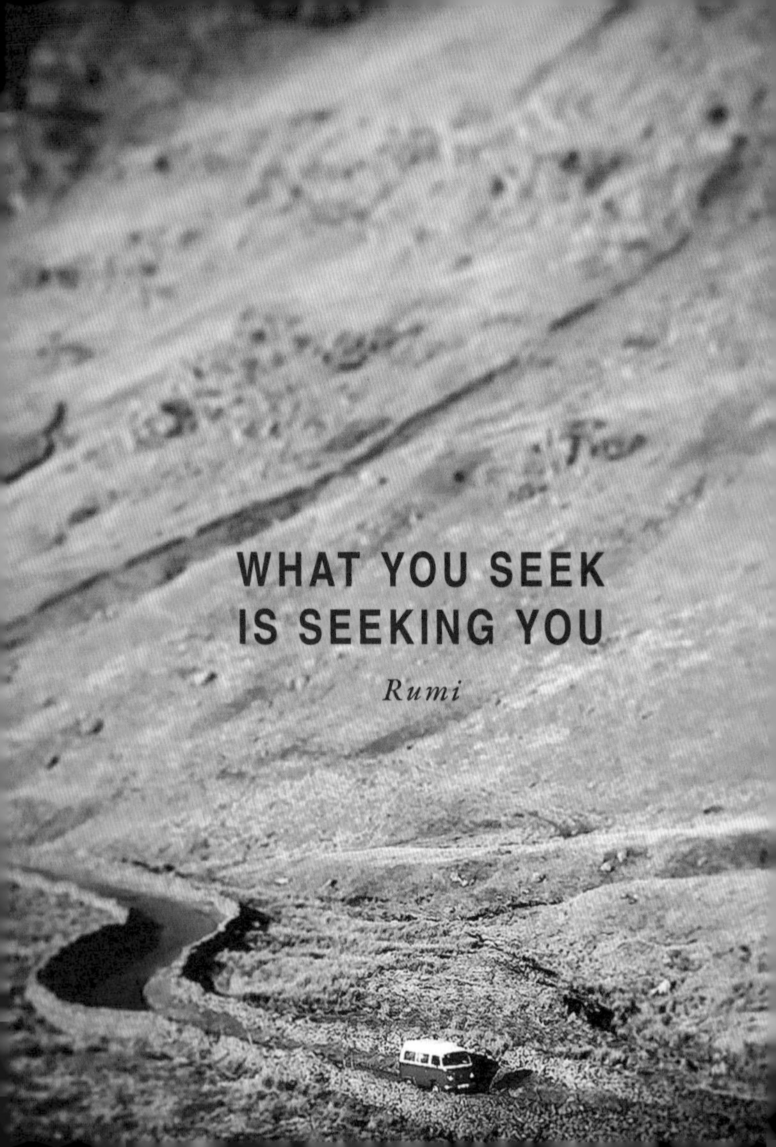

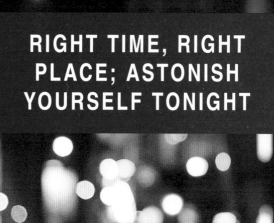

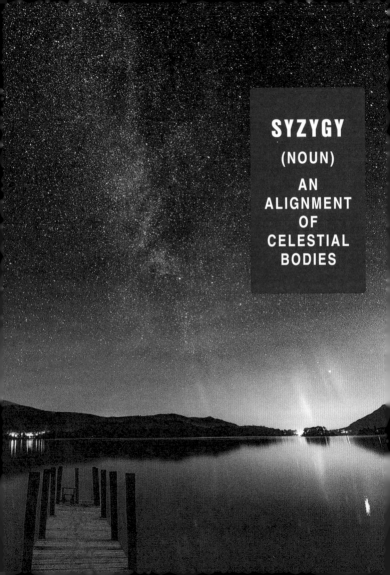

SYZYGY

(NOUN)

AN ALIGNMENT OF CELESTIAL BODIES

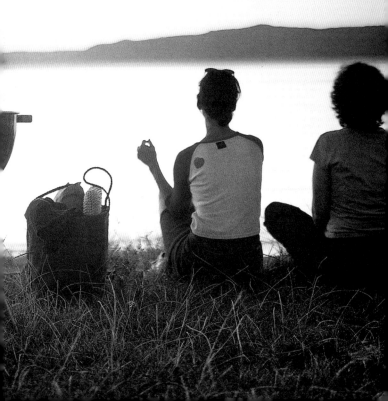

EMBRACE THE POWER OF THE EVENING SKY

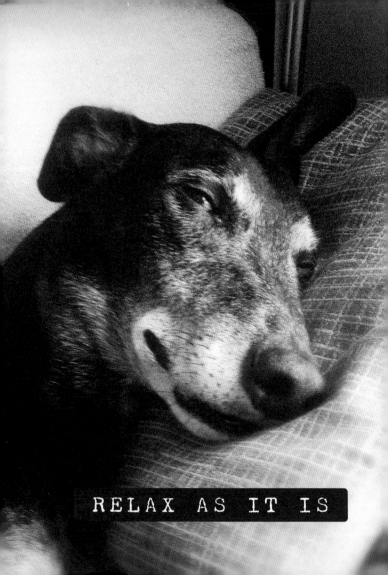

RELAX AS IT IS

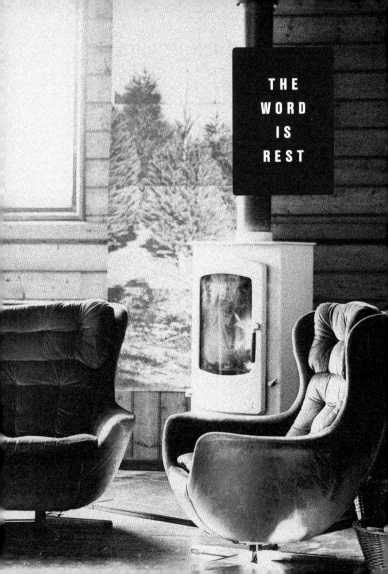

THE
WORD
IS
REST

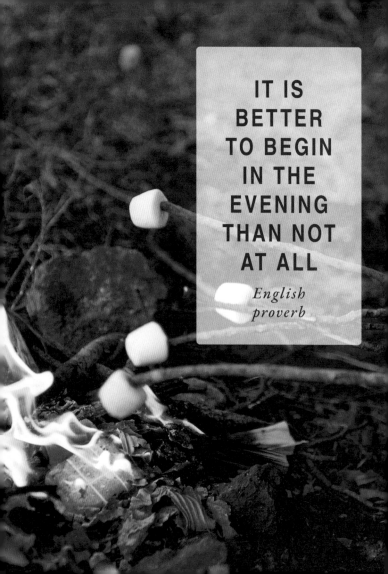

IT IS BETTER TO BEGIN IN THE EVENING THAN NOT AT ALL

English proverb

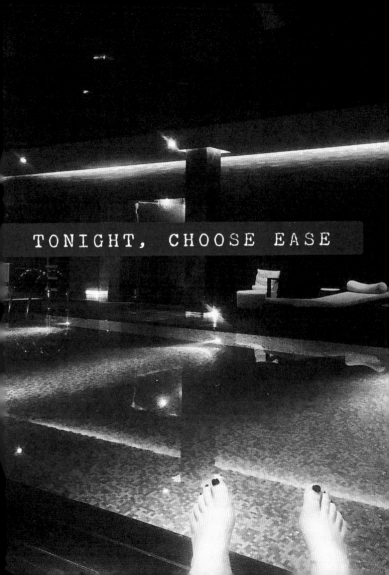

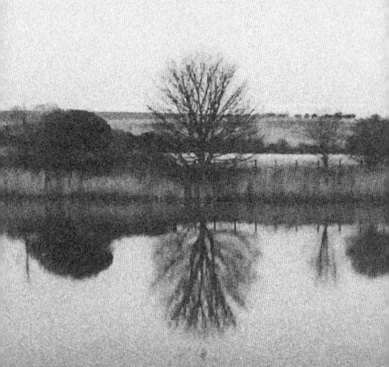

TO THE MIND THAT IS STILL,
THE WHOLE UNIVERSE SURRENDERS

Lao Tzu

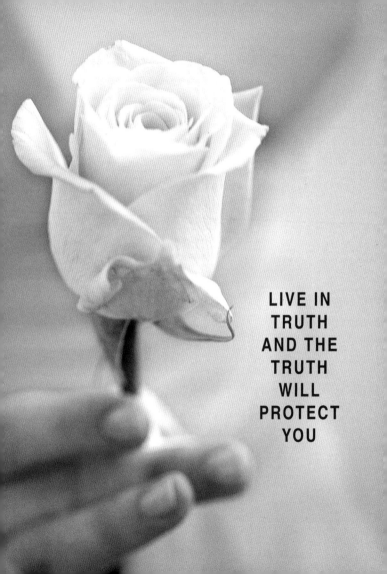

LIVE IN
TRUTH
AND THE
TRUTH
WILL
PROTECT
YOU

ANTICIPATE THE DIFFICULT BY MANAGING THE EASY

Lao Tzu

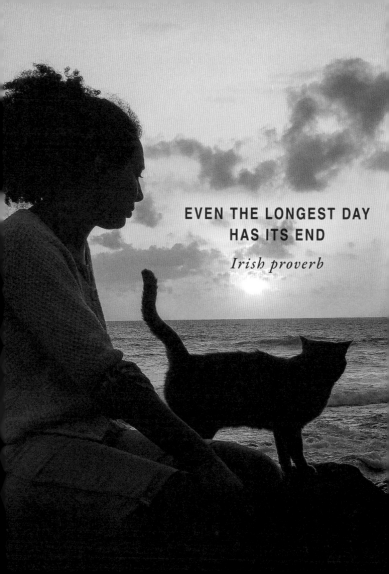

EVEN THE LONGEST DAY
HAS ITS END

Irish proverb

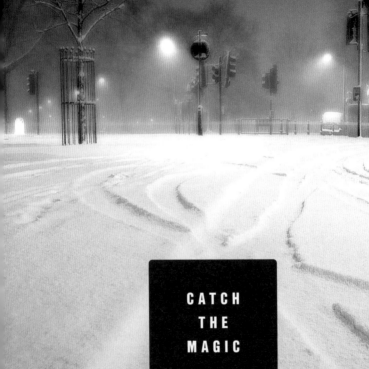

CATCH
THE
MAGIC

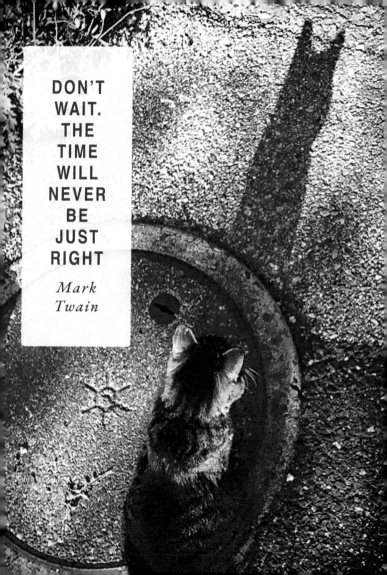

DON'T
WAIT.
THE
TIME
WILL
NEVER
BE
JUST
RIGHT

*Mark
Twain*

Thousands of candles

can be lighted from

a single candle, and

the life of the candle

will not be shortened.

Happiness never decrease:

by being shared

Buddha

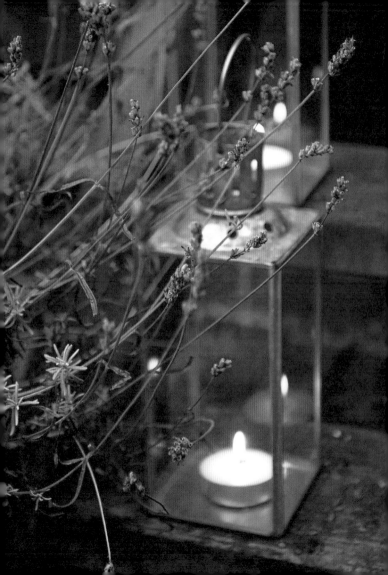

A BEAUTIFUL SUNSET THAT
WAS MISTAKEN FOR A DAWN

Claude Debussy

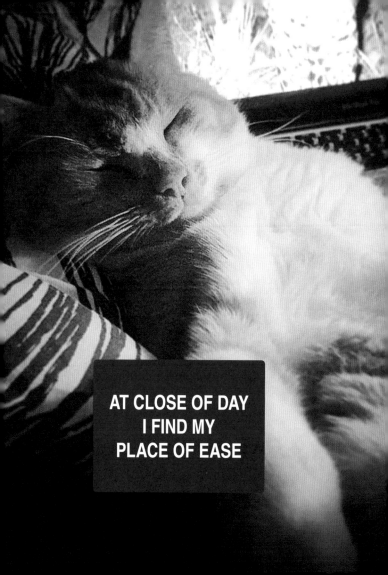

AT CLOSE OF DAY
I FIND MY
PLACE OF EASE

THE ONLY
MIRACLES
THAT CAN'T REACH YOU
ARE THE ONES
YOU WAIT
AROUND FOR

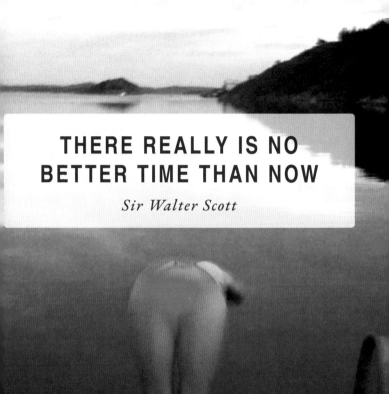

THERE REALLY IS NO BETTER TIME THAN NOW

Sir Walter Scott

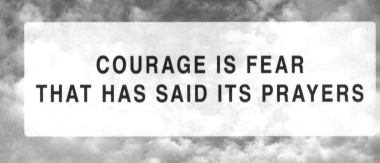

**COURAGE IS FEAR
THAT HAS SAID ITS PRAYERS**

MY SUN SETS TO RISE AGAIN

Robert Browning

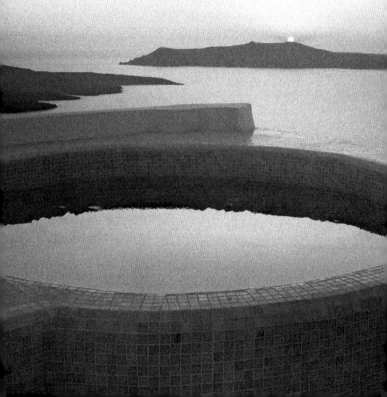

Silence

is a source

of great

strength

Lao Tzu

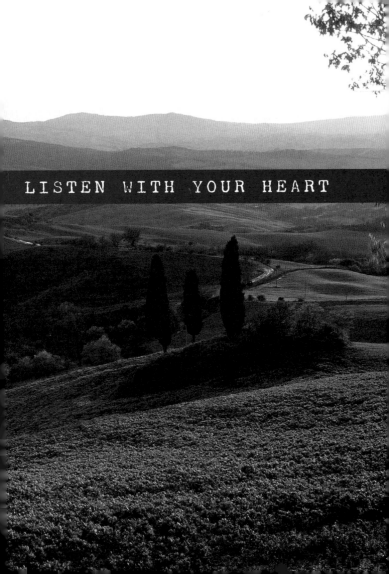

LISTEN WITH YOUR HEART

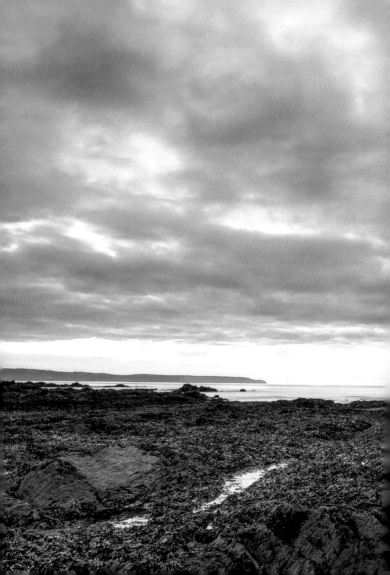

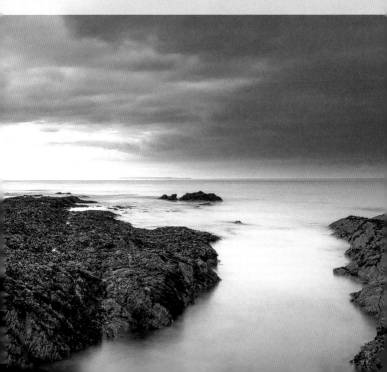

THERE'S NO BETTER SOUND TO HEAR
THAN THE OCEAN, THE WIND, AND THE
RAIN ALL AT ONCE, LATE AT NIGHT

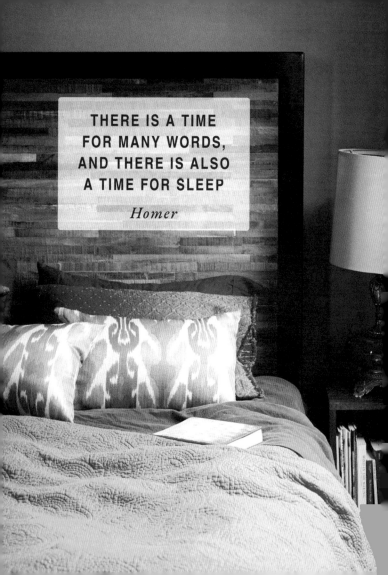

THERE IS A TIME
FOR MANY WORDS,
AND THERE IS ALSO
A TIME FOR SLEEP

Homer

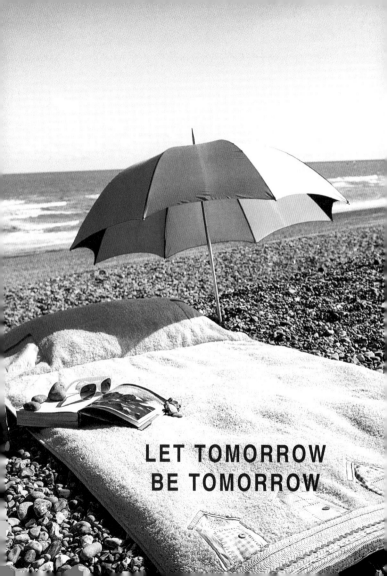

LET TOMORROW
BE TOMORROW

WHAT LIES BEHIND YOU AND WHAT LIES IN FRONT OF YOU PALES IN COMPARISON TO WHAT LIES INSIDE OF YOU

Ralph Waldo Emerson

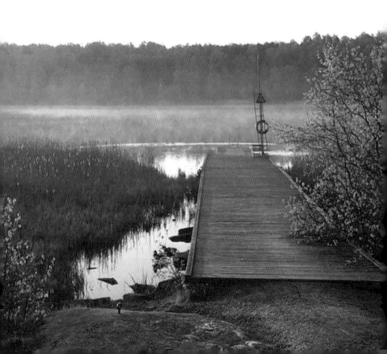

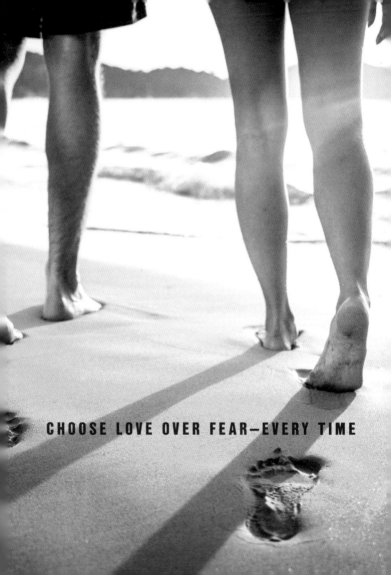

CHOOSE LOVE OVER FEAR—EVERY TIME

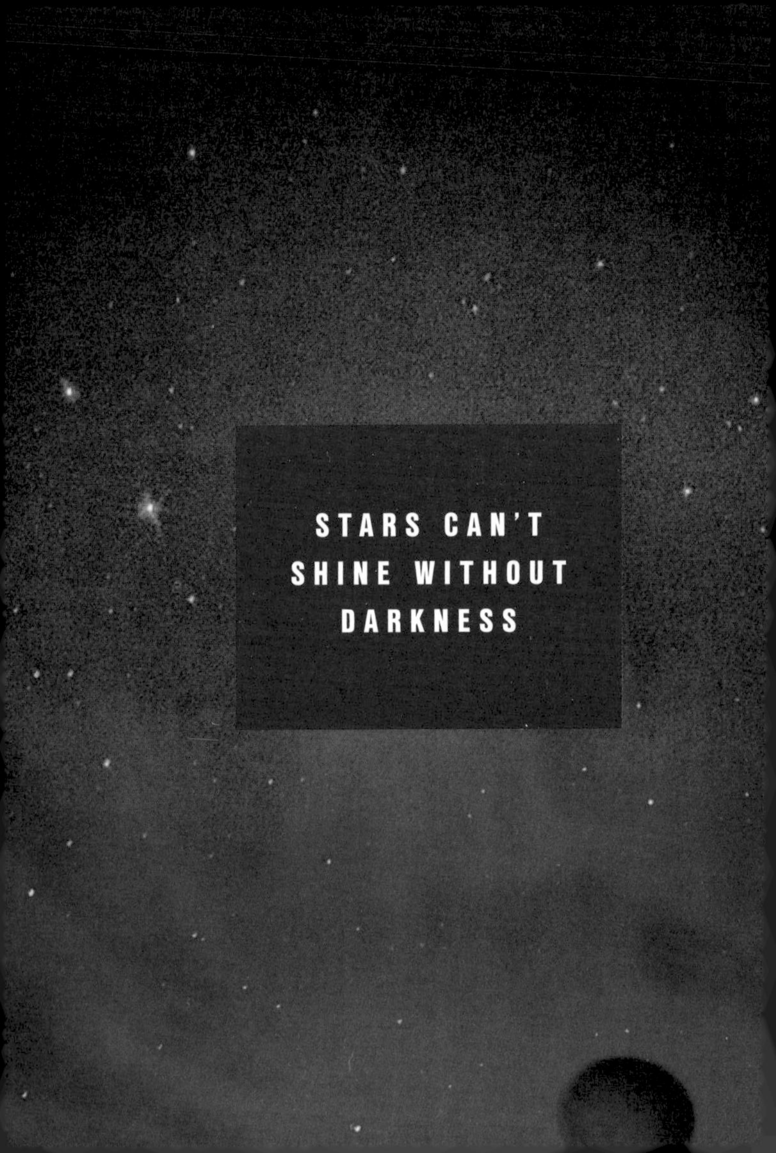

STARS CAN'T
SHINE WITHOUT
DARKNESS

FROM REALLY FAR
OUT IN SPACE
DO YOU KNOW WHAT
YOU LOOK LIKE?
A SUPER STAR

IT DOES NOT
REQUIRE MANY WORDS
TO SPEAK
THE TRUTH

Chief Joseph

HONOR THE STILLNESS

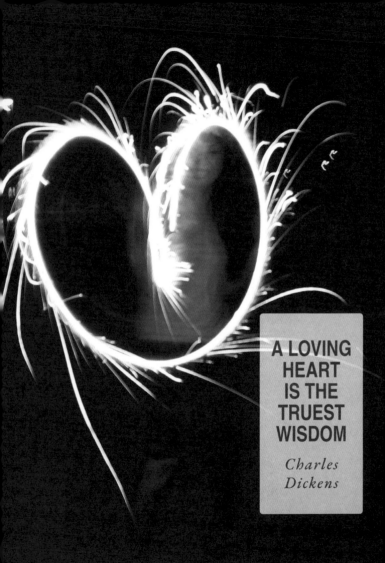

A LOVING
HEART
IS THE
TRUEST
WISDOM

*Charles
Dickens*

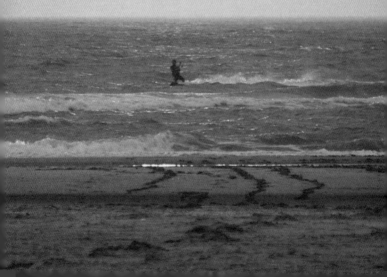

LET THE BEAUTY OF WHAT
YOU LOVE BE WHAT YOU DO

Rumi

YOU DON'T HAVE TO REACH FOR THE STARS, THEY ARE ALREADY WITHIN YOU

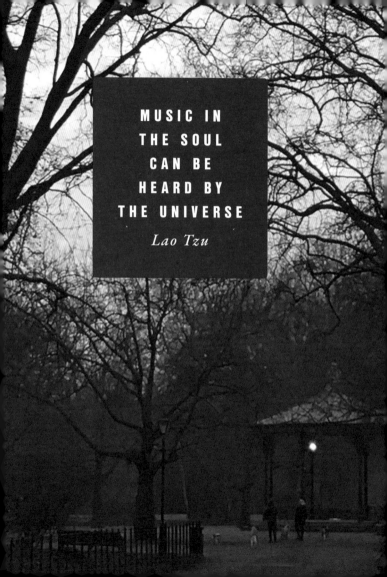

MUSIC IN
THE SOUL
CAN BE
HEARD BY
THE UNIVERSE

Lao Tzu

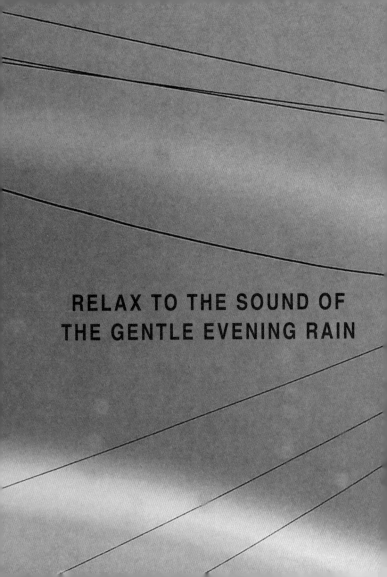

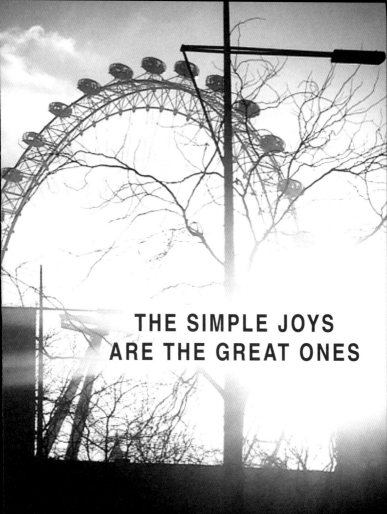

THE SIMPLE JOYS
ARE THE GREAT ONES

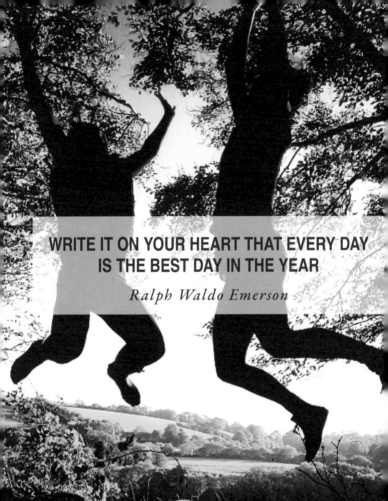

WRITE IT ON YOUR HEART THAT EVERY DAY
IS THE BEST DAY IN THE YEAR

Ralph Waldo Emerson

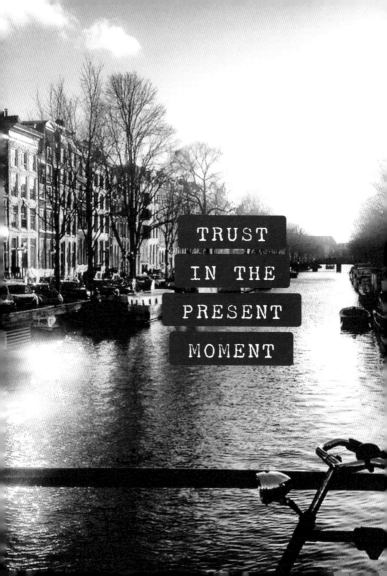

TRUST
IN THE
PRESENT
MOMENT

No act of kindness,
no matter how small,
is ever wasted

Aesop

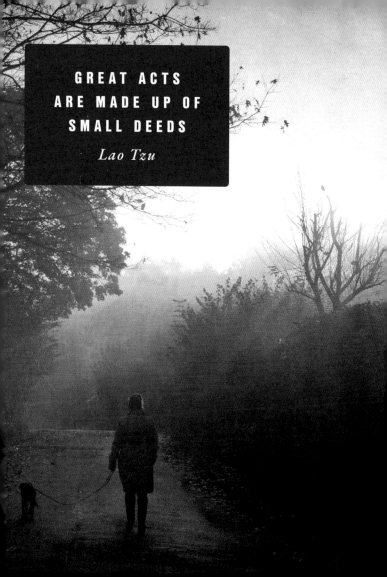

GREAT ACTS
ARE MADE UP OF
SMALL DEEDS

Lao Tzu

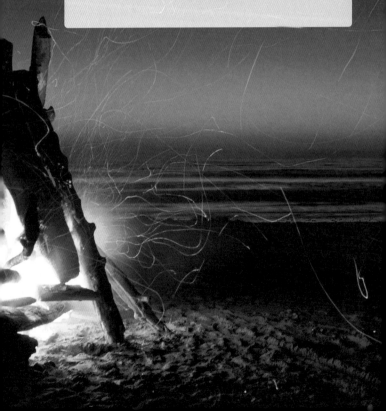

I'VE LOVED THE STARS
TOO FONDLY TO BE
FEARFUL OF THE NIGHT

Galileo

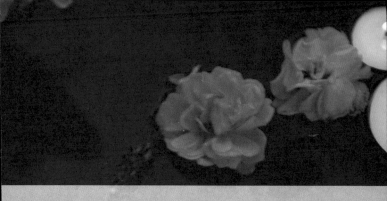

MY GUIDING WORD IS SERENITY

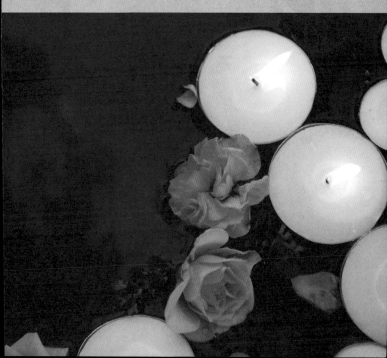

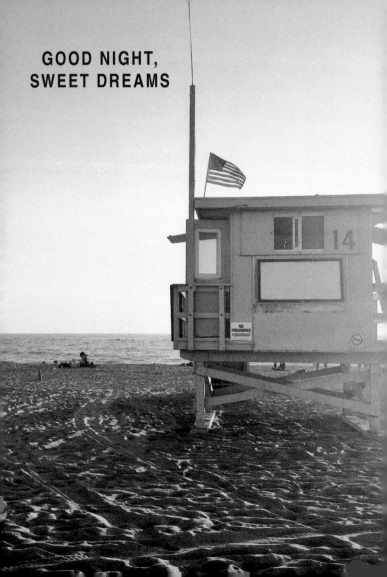

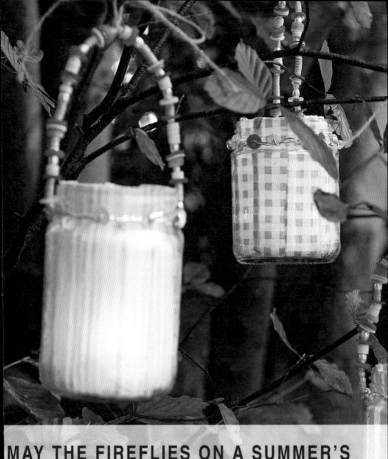

MAY THE FIREFLIES ON A SUMMER'S
EVE LIGHT UP YOUR PATH

AND REMEMBER, NO MATTER WHERE YOU GO, THERE YOU ARE

Confucius

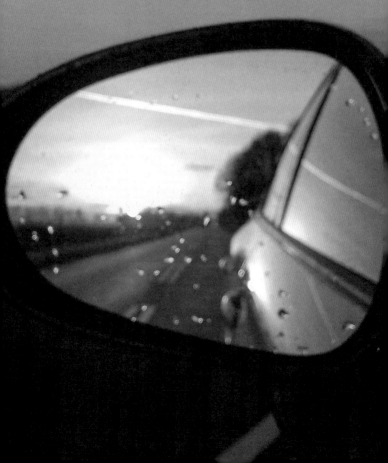

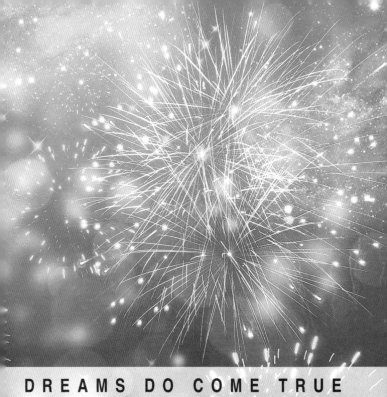

DREAMS DO COME TRUE

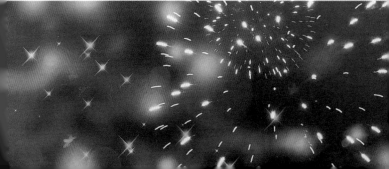

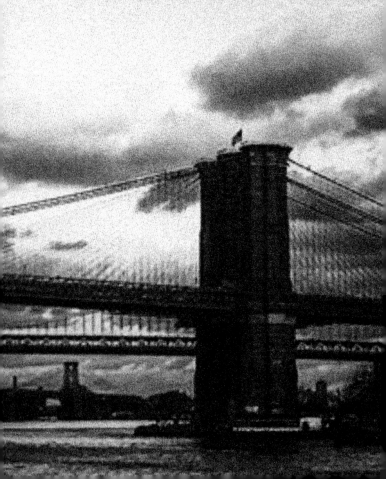

TOMORROW AWAITS

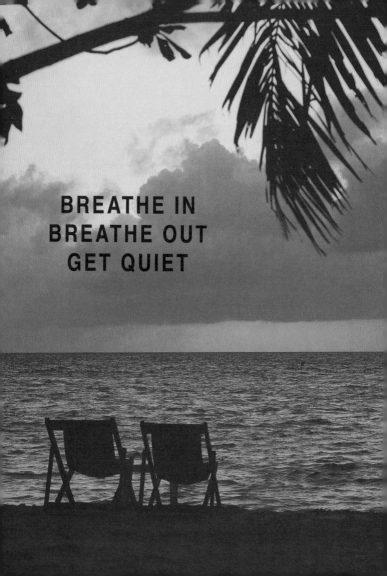

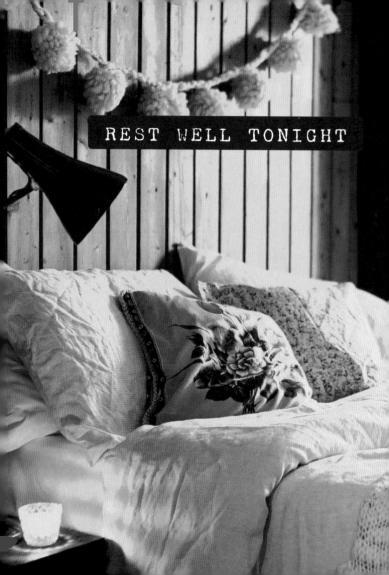

REST WELL TONIGHT

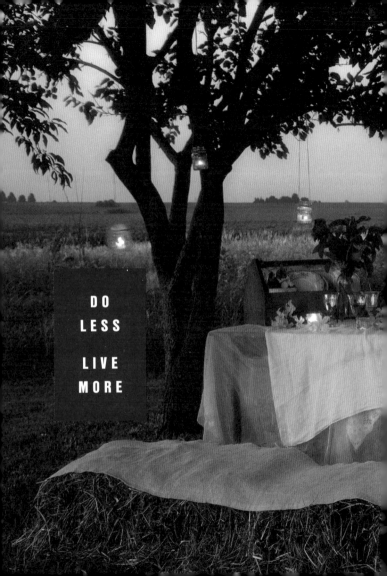

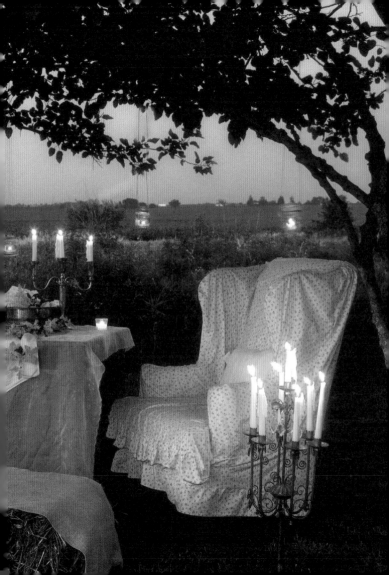

THE BEST PREPARATION FOR TOMORROW IS TO DO TODAY'S WORK SUPERBLY WELL

William Osler

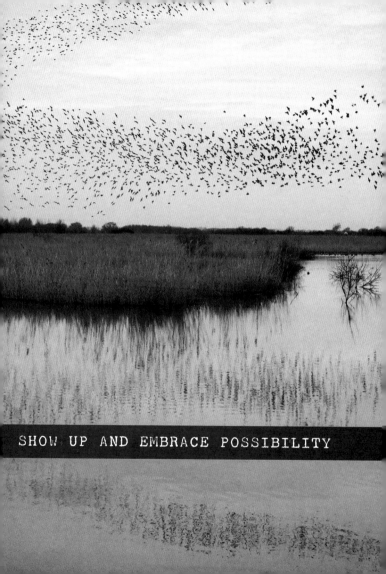

SHOW UP AND EMBRACE POSSIBILITY

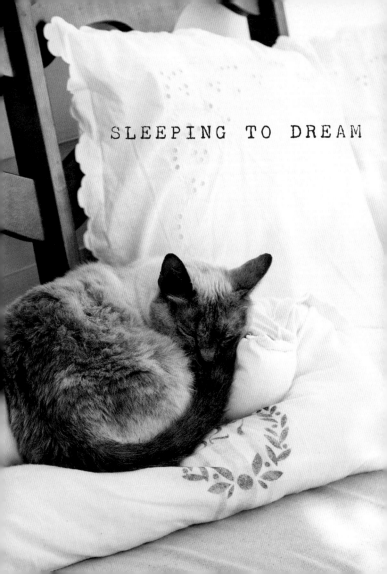

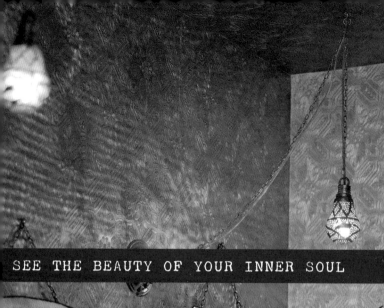

SEE THE BEAUTY OF YOUR INNER SOUL

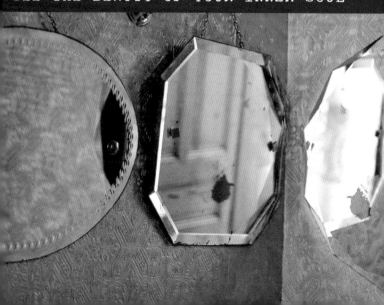

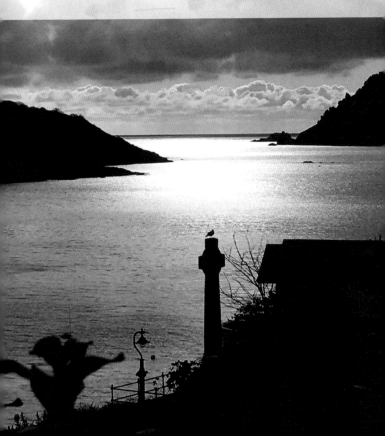

IT IS ONLY THROUGH SHADOWS
THAT ONE COMES TO KNOW THE LIGHT

Saint Catherine of Siena

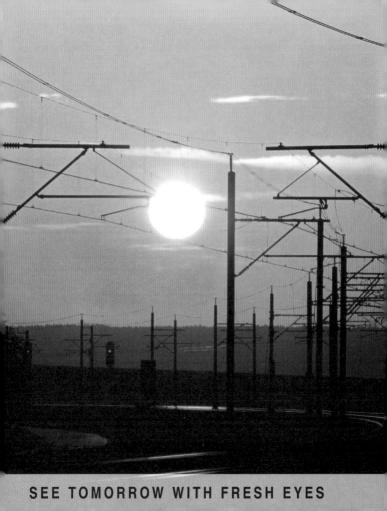

SEE TOMORROW WITH FRESH EYES

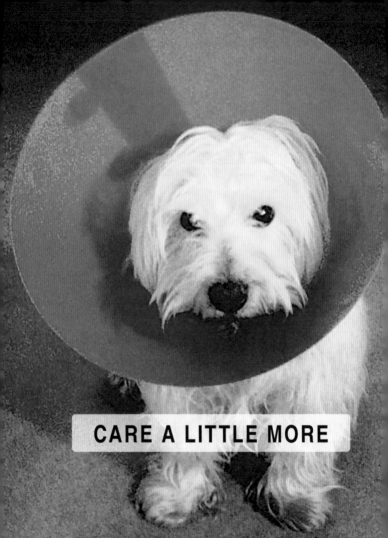

CARE A LITTLE MORE

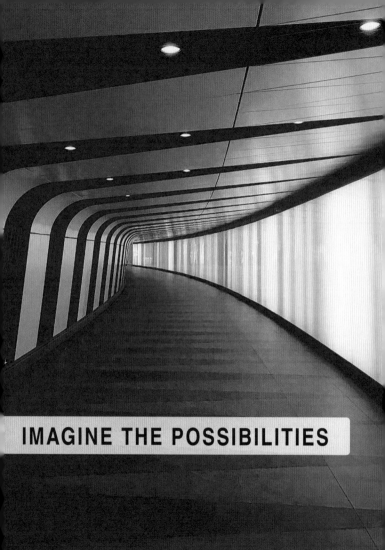

IMAGINE THE POSSIBILITIES

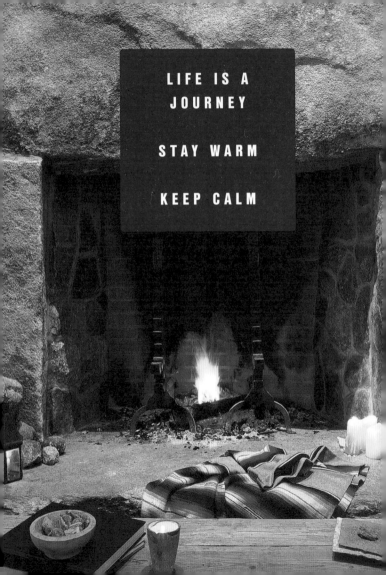

SLEEP
DREAM
BELIEVE

EVEN IF I KNEW THAT TOMORROW
THE WORLD WOULD GO TO PIECES,
I WOULD STILL PLANT MY APPLE TREE

Martin Luther

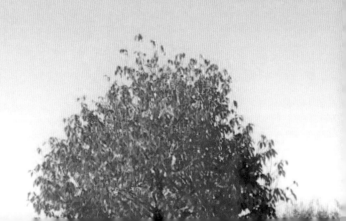

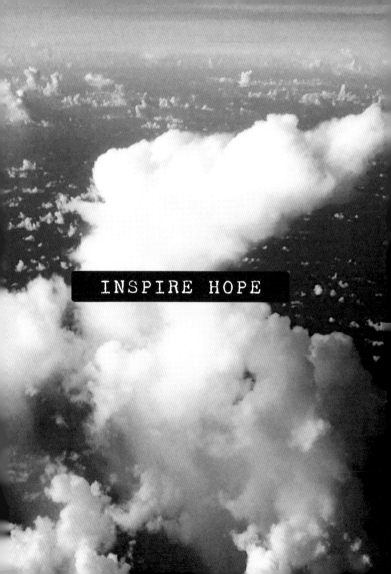

INSPIRE HOPE

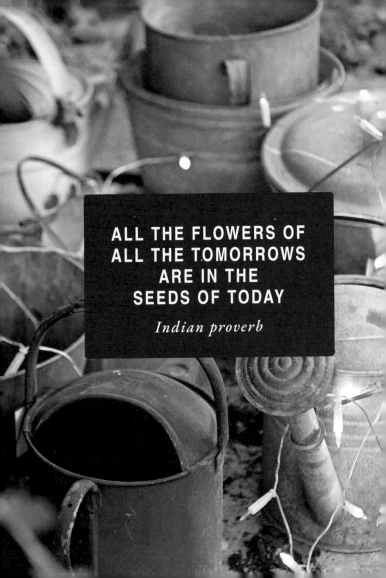

ALL THE FLOWERS OF
ALL THE TOMORROWS
ARE IN THE
SEEDS OF TODAY

Indian proverb

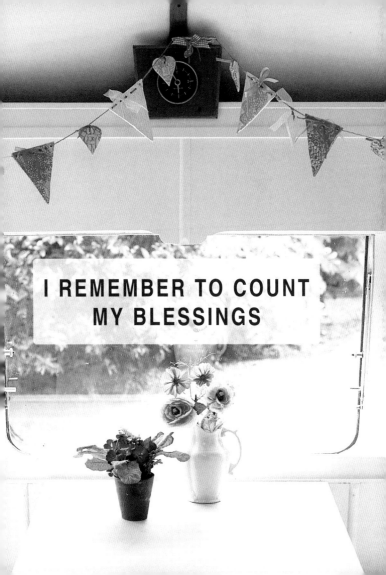

THE FUTURE IS NO MORE UNCERTAIN THAN THE PRESENT

Walt Whitman

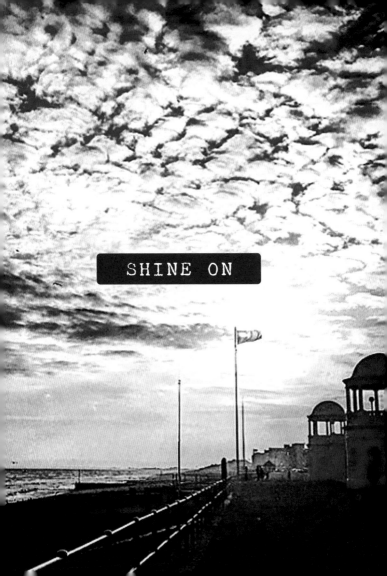

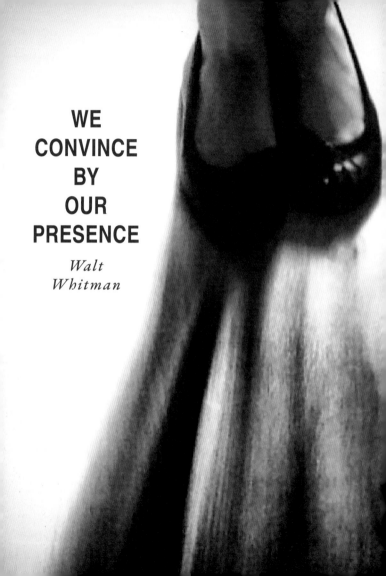

**WE
CONVINCE
BY
OUR
PRESENCE**

*Walt
Whitman*

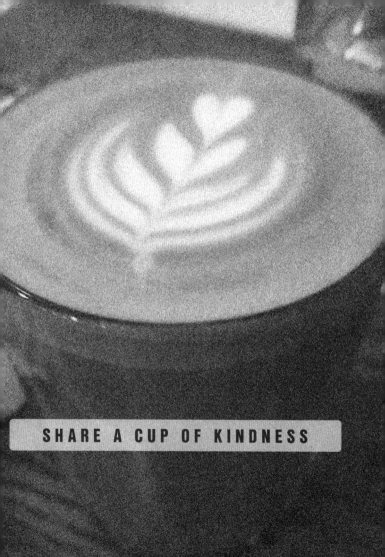

SHARE A CUP OF KINDNESS

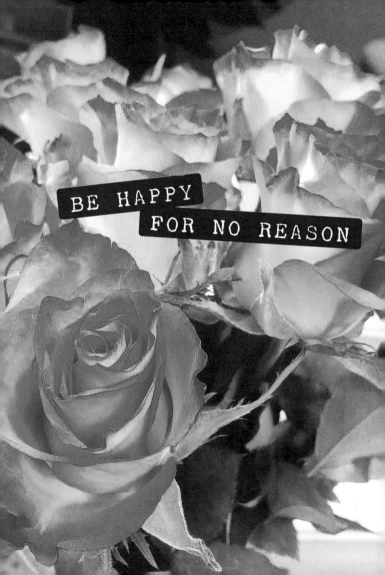

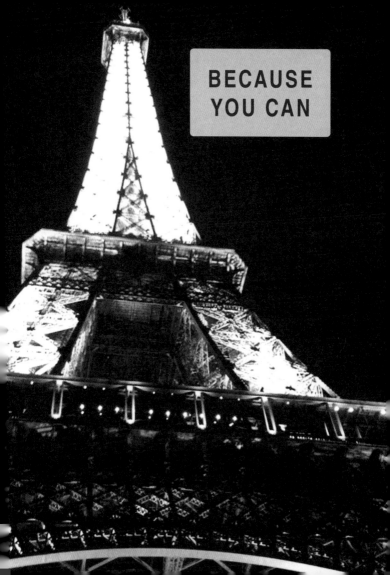

KEEP IT SIMPLE

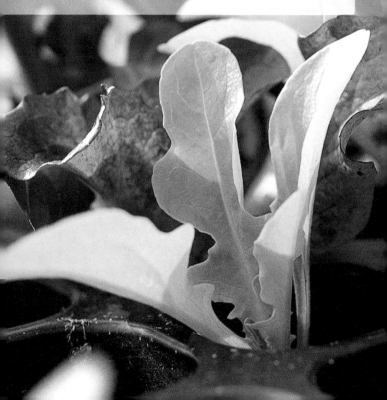

NATURE DOES NOT HURRY,
YET EVERYTHING IS ACCOMPLISHED

Lao Tzu

OH, THE SUMMER NIGHT,
HAS A SMILE OF LIGHT,
AND SHE SITS ON
A SAPPHIRE THRONE

Byron Procter

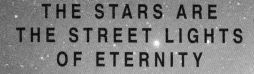

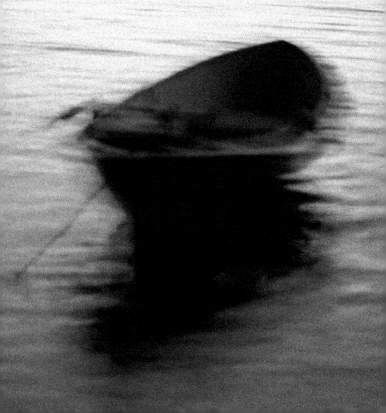

KNOWLEDGE COMES,
BUT WISDOM LINGERS

Alfred, Lord Tennyson

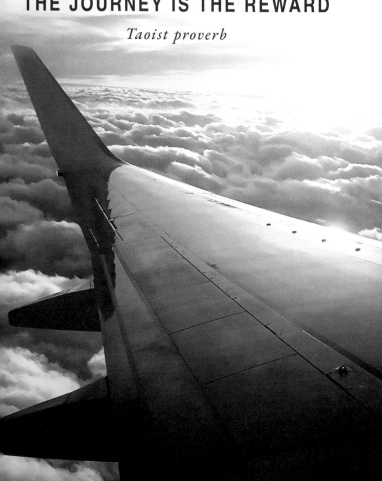

THE JOURNEY IS THE REWARD

Taoist proverb

NO

SNOWFLAKE

EVER

FALLS

IN

THE

WRONG

PLACE

Zen proverb

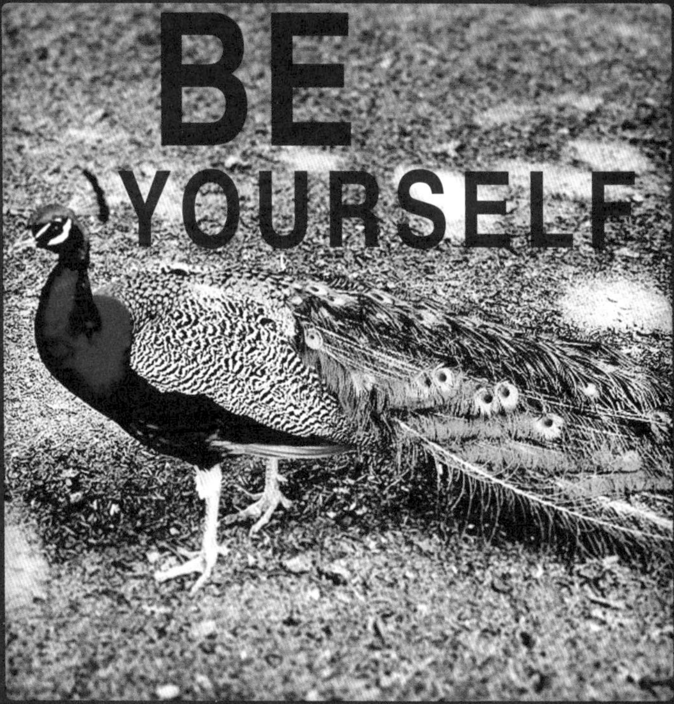
BE
YOURSELF

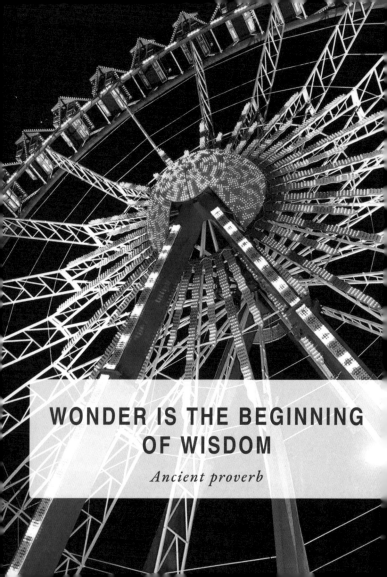

WONDER IS THE BEGINNING
OF WISDOM

Ancient proverb

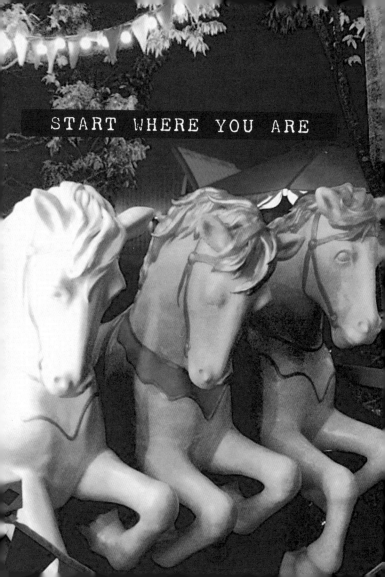

START WHERE YOU ARE

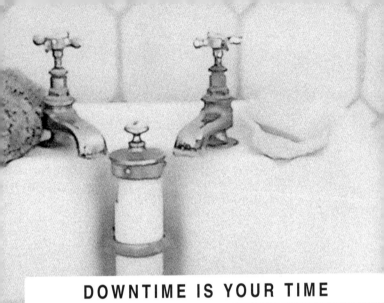

DOWNTIME IS YOUR TIME

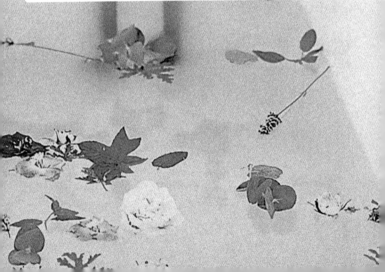

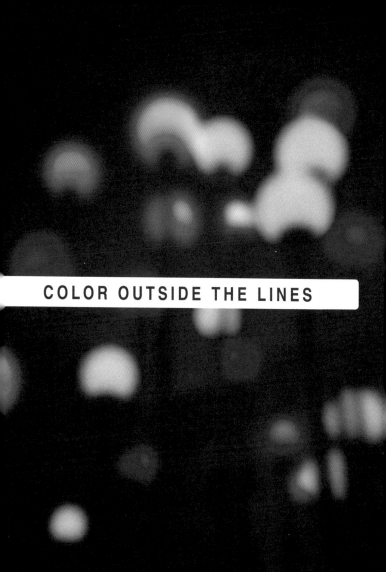

COLOR OUTSIDE THE LINES

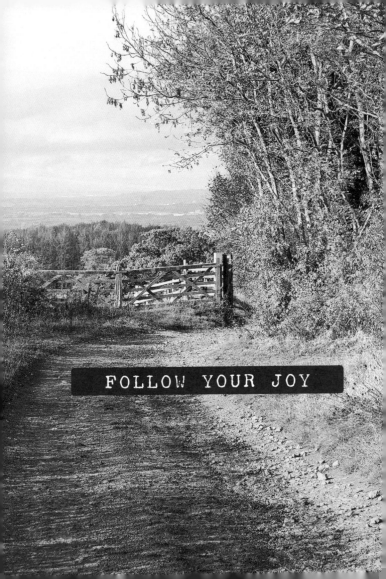

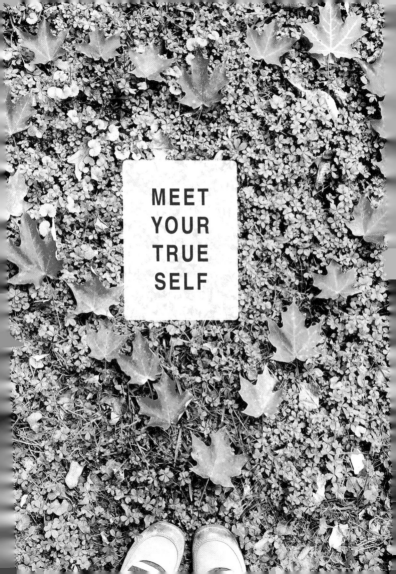

TO ALL, TO EACH, A FAIR GOOD NIGHT,
AND PLEASING DREAMS, AND
SLUMBERS LIGHT

Sir Walter Scott

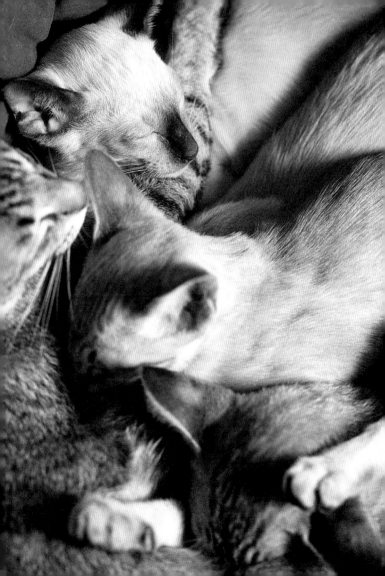

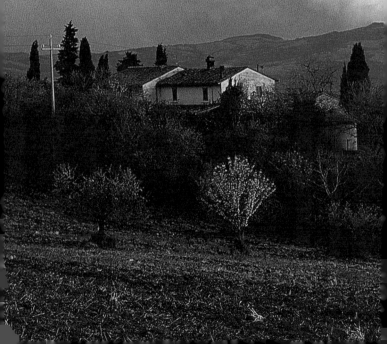

THE SETTING SUN OFFERS
AN INVITATION TO WONDER

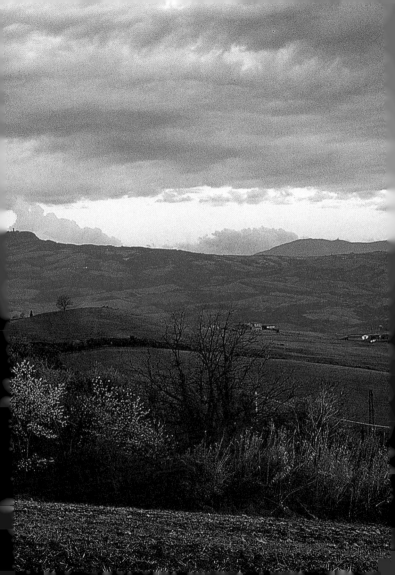

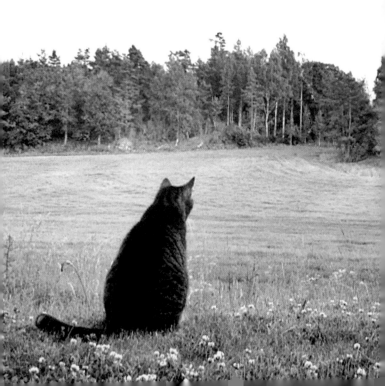

BE CURIOUS

THE GREATEST MIRACLE OF ALL IS FOUND IN WHAT IS MOST ORDINARY

THE SUN
WILL NOT RISE
OR SET
WITHOUT
MY NOTICE,
AND THANKS

Winslow Homer

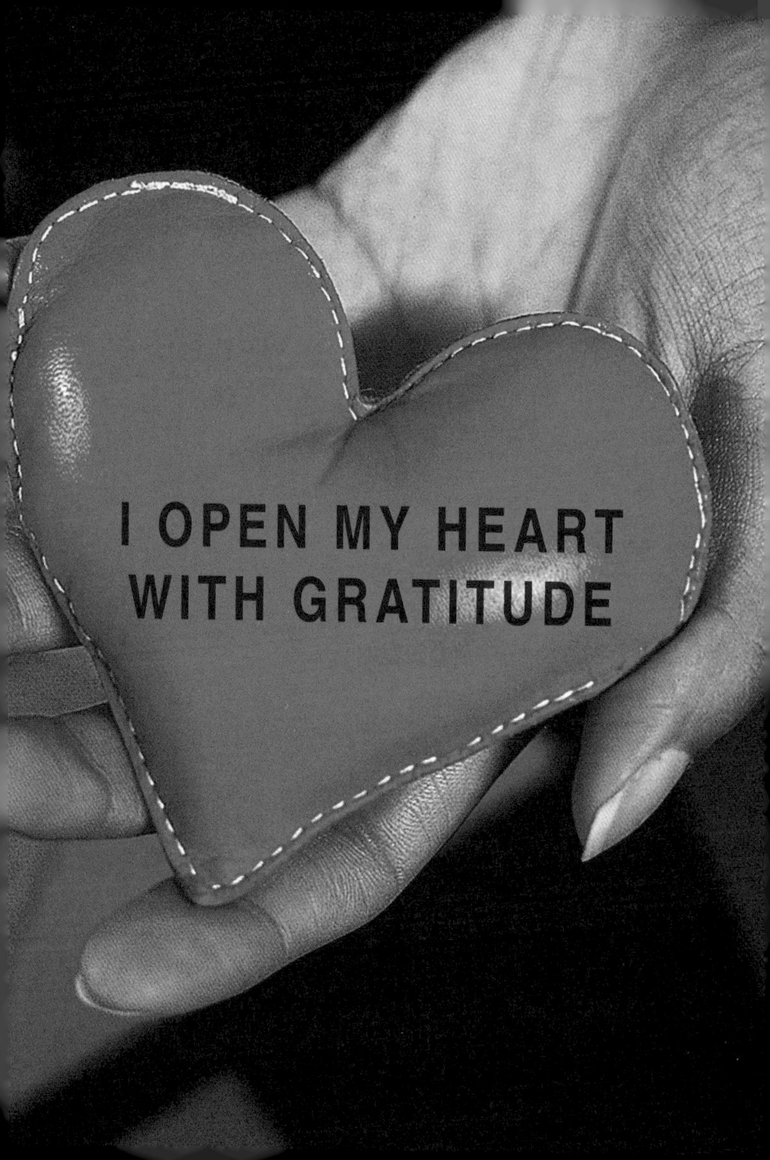
I OPEN MY HEART
WITH GRATITUDE

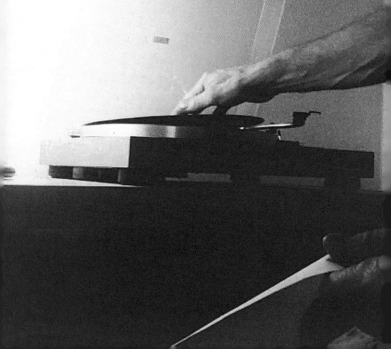

**THERE IS GUIDANCE
FOR EACH OF US, AND
BY LOVELY LISTENING,
WE SHALL HEAR
THE RIGHT WORD**

Ralph Waldo Emerson

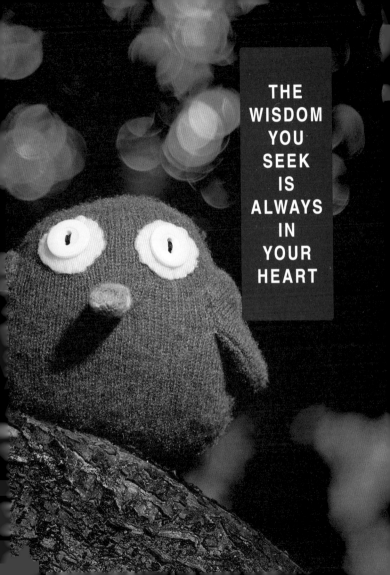

THE
WISDOM
YOU
SEEK
IS
ALWAYS
IN
YOUR
HEART

YOU HAVE NOT LIVED TODAY UNTIL YOU
HAVE DONE SOMETHING FOR SOMEONE
WHO CAN NEVER REPAY YOU

John Bunyan

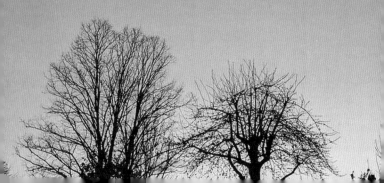

THREE THINGS
CANNOT BE
LONG HIDDEN:
THE SUN,
THE MOON,
AND
THE TRUTH

Buddha

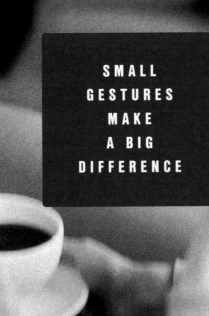

SMALL
GESTURES
MAKE
A BIG
DIFFERENCE

TO BE IS TO DO

Immanuel Kant

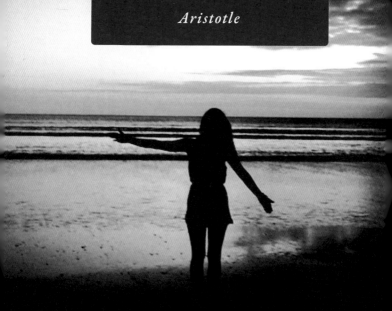

HAPPINESS DEPENDS UPON OURSELVES

Aristotle

IT'S NOT WHAT
HAPPENS TO YOU,
BUT HOW YOU
REACT TO IT
THAT MATTERS

Epictetus

I AM
AT HOME
IN THE
WORLD

PICTURE CREDITS

Key: **ph** = photographer

Front cover © Ryland Peters and Small/Styled by Selina Lake at her home. **ph** Debi Treloar; **back cover** © Ryland Peters and Small/**ph** Peter Cassidy; **page 1** © Ryland Peters and Small/ www.helenbratby.co.uk. **ph** Debi Treloar; **pages 2–3** Getty/© Landscapes by Kris Williams; **page 4** © Tia Lovisa; follow her on Instagram: @tltraveler; **page 6** © Therese Oertenblad: follow her on Instagram @thessan_11; **page 7** Getty/© AROON PHUKEED; **page 9** © Megan Winter-Barker: follow her on Instagram @megwinterbarker; **page 10** Getty/© vetas; **page 11** Getty/© Jason Cameron; **page 13** © Ryland Peters and Small/**ph** Claire Richardson; **page 14** © CICO Books/**ph** Simon Brown; **page 17** Getty/© Edd Lange/EyeEm; **page 18** © Zia Mattocks; **page 20** © Ryland Peters and Small/**ph** William Shaw; **page 21** © Zia Mattocks; **page 23** © Susan Waller; **page 24** Getty/© Landscapes by Kris Williams; **page 25** Getty/© beppeverge; **page 26** © Ryland Peters and Small/**ph** Debi Treloar; **page 27** © Lena Karlsson: follow her on Instagram @asakapop or check out her website: www.asakapop.com; **page 29** © Ryland Peters and Small/**ph** Claire Richardson; **page 30** © Lucy Jackson: follow her on Instagram @bugjackson; **page 31** © CICO Books/**ph** Claire Richardson; **page 32** © Ryland Peters and Small/Styled by Selina Lake at her home. **ph** Debi Treloar; **page 33** © Ryland Peters and Small/The home of Fifi Mandirac in Paris. **ph** Debi Treloar; **page 35** © Ryland Peters and Small/**ph** Chris Tubbs; **page 36** © Megan Winter-Barker: follow her on Instagram @megwinterbarker; **page 37** Getty/© Caiaimage/Tom Merton; **page 38** Getty/© john finney photography; **page 39** © Ryland Peters and Small/**ph** Ian Wallace; **page 40** © Paul Tilby (paultilby.com); **page 41** © Ryland Peters and Small/www.vintagevacations.co.uk. **ph** Debi Treloar; **page 42** © Ryland Peters and Small/www.lovelanecaravans.com. **ph** Debi Treloar; **page 43** © Lucy Jackson: follow her on Instagram @bugjackson; **page 44** © Lucy Jackson: follow her on Instagram @bugjackson; **page 45** © Ryland Peters and Small/**ph** Winfried Heinze; **page 47** © Paul Tilby (paultilby.com); **page 48** Getty/© Hair Fashion; **page 49** © Lena Karlsson: follow her on Instagram @asakapop or check out her website: www.asakapop.com; **page 51** © Ryland Peters and Small/**ph** Debi Treloar; **page 52** © Lena Karlsson: follow her on Instagram @asakapop or check out her website: www.asakapop.com; **page 53** © Megan Winter-Barker: follow her on Instagram @megwinterbarker; **page 55** © Lena Karlsson: follow her on Instagram @asakapop or check out her website: www.asakapop.com; **page 56** © Lena Karlsson: follow her on Instagram @asakapop or check out her website: www.asakapop.com; **page 57** © CICO Books/**ph** Mark Scott; **page 59** © Ryland Peters and Small/**ph** Peter Cassidy; **pages 60–61** Getty/© Rob Maynard; **page 62** © Ryland Peters and Small/The home of Jonathan Sela & Megan Schoenbachler. **ph** Catherine Gratwicke; **page 63** © CICO Books/ **ph** Claire Richardson; **page 64** © Lena Karlsson: follow her on Instagram @asakapop or check out her website: www.asakapop.com; **page 65** Getty/© oneinchpunch; **page 66** © Emma Kirkby: follow her on Instagram @emmaloukirkby; **page 69** © Tia Lovisa; follow her on Instagram: @tltraveler; **page 70** Getty/© Kazuo Yasuoka/EyeEm; **page 71** Getty/© Lars

Boonstra/EyeEm; **page 73** © Zia Mattocks; **page 74** © Emma Kirkby: follow her on Instagram @emmaloukirkby; **page 75** © Lucy Jackson: follow her on Instagram @bugjackson; **page 76** © Rebecca Langston; follow her on Instagram: @bexlang; **page 77** © Rebecca Langston; follow her on Instagram: @bexlang; **page 79** Getty/© Dirk Wüstenhagen Imagery; **page 80** Getty/© Lijuan Guo Photography; **page 81** © Ryland Peters and Small/**ph** Debi Treloar; **page 82** Getty/© Ailbhe O'Donnell; **page 83** © CICO Books/**ph** Claire Richardson; **page 84** Getty/© Coco Gubbels/EyeEm; **page 85** Getty/© 8213erika; **page 86** © Megan Winter-Barker: follow her on Instagram @megwinterbarker; **page 87** © Emma Kirkby: follow her on Instagram @emmaloukirkby; **page 88** Getty/© Alessandro Bolis; **page 89** © Ryland Peters and Small/www.vintagevacations.co.uk. ph Debi Treloar; **pages 90–91** © CICO Books/**ph** Mark Lohman; **page 93** Getty/© Mint Images; **page 94** © CICO Books/**ph** Mark Lohman; **page 95** © Ryland Peters and Small/The restaurant "Derriere" designed and owned by the "Hazouz Brothers". **ph** Debi Treloar; **page 96** © Zia Mattocks; **page 97** Getty/© Coco Gubbels/EyeEm; **page 98** © Emma Kirkby: follow her on Instagram @emmaloukirkby; **page 99** © Anna Galkina; follow her on Instagram: @wolflick; **page 100** © Ryland Peters and Small/A cottage in Connecticut designed by Benard M. Wharton. **ph** Chris Tubbs; **page 102** © Lucy Jackson: follow her on Instagram @bugjackson; **page 103** © Lena Karlsson: follow her on Instagram @asakapop or check out her website: www.asakapop.com; **page 104** © Ryland Peters and Small/**ph** Debi Treloar; **page 105** © CICO Books/**ph** Claire Richardson; **page 107** © Rebecca Langston; follow her on Instagram: @bexlang; **page 108** © Emma Kirkby: follow her on Instagram @emmaloukirkby; **page 109** © Emma Kirkby: follow her on Instagram @emmaloukirkby; **page 110** © Emma Kirkby: follow her on Instagram @emmaloukirkby; **page 111** © Lena Karlsson: follow her on Instagram @asakapop or check out her website: www.asakapop.com; **page 113** © Ryland Peters and Small/**ph** Caroline Hughes; **page 115** Getty/© Hugo; **page 116** © Ryland Peters and Small/**ph** Jan Baldwin; **page 117** © Antony De Rienzo; follow him on Instagram: @antonyderienzo; **page 119** © Emma Kirkby: follow her on Instagram @emmaloukirkby; **page 120** © Tia Lovisa; follow her on Instagram: @tltraveler; **page 121** © Lena Karlsson: follow her on Instagram @asakapop or check out her website: www.asakapop.com; **page 122** © Ryland Peters and Small/**ph** William Lingwood; **page 123** © Lena Karlsson: follow her on Instagram @asakapop or check out her website: www.asakapop.com; **page 124** © Ryland Peters and Small/**ph** Steve Painter; **page 125** Getty/© Cyndi Monaghan; **page 127** © Ryland Peters and Small/**ph** Andrew Wood; **pages 128–129** © Ryland Peters and Small/**ph** Peter Cassidy; **page 130** © Lena Karlsson: follow her on Instagram @asakapop or check out her website: www.asakapop.com; **page 132** © Antony De Rienzo; follow him on Instagram: @antonyderienzo; **page 133** © Ryland Peters and Small/**ph** Claire Richardson; **page 134** © Lena Karlsson: follow her on Instagram: @asakapop or check out her website: www.asakapop.com; **page 135** © CICO Books/**ph** Geoff Dann; **page 137** © Simon Jackson; follow him on Instagram: @indys_shots; **page 138** © Ryland Peters and Small/**ph** Debi Treloar; **page 139** © Emma Kirkby: follow her on Instagram @emmaloukirkby; **page 140** © Hannah Styles; follow her on Instagram: @hanstyl3s; **page 142** © Paul Tilby (paultilby.com)